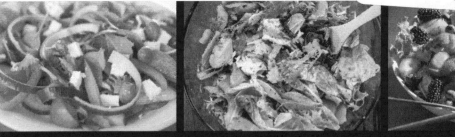

TOXIC SUPERFOODS COOKBOOK

275 Recipes Inspired by Sally K. Norton to Detoxify your Diets and Safeguard Your Body

Lily Mae Parker

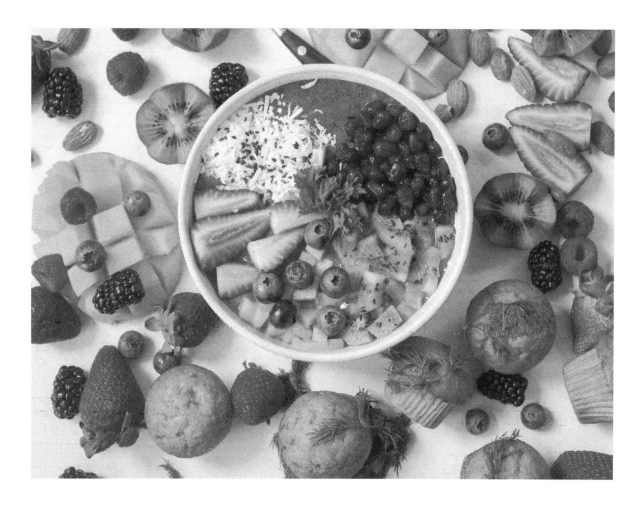

Table of Contents

Introduction: The Hidden Danger in Your Healthy Diet

Imagine this: You've spent years doing everything "right" for your health. You fill your grocery cart with organic spinach, snack on almonds, and swap your regular fries for baked sweet potatoes. Your pantry is stocked with the latest superfoods that everyone swears by—chia seeds, kale, and green smoothies. On paper, you're the picture of healthy living. So why do you still feel exhausted, bloated, and in pain? Why are you battling brain fog, joint stiffness, and mysterious chronic ailments that no doctor seems to explain? That was me. For years, I followed a plant-heavy, clean-eating lifestyle because it was supposed to be the key to vibrant health. I had every reason to believe I was nourishing my body, but instead, I was becoming sicker. Inflammation, fatigue, and anxiety were my constant companions. My joints ached, my digestion was a mess, and I was perpetually tired. Worse, I couldn't figure out why.

The turning point came when I stumbled upon a hidden truth about the very foods I thought were healing me. The problem wasn't a lack of healthy choices. The problem was toxicity—and it was coming from those same "superfoods" I had relied on for years. Spinach, almonds, sweet potatoes, and other beloved plant foods were loaded with oxalates—natural compounds that can wreak havoc on your body when consumed in excess. Oxalates were quietly accumulating in my system, triggering all the symptoms I'd been fighting for so long.

It wasn't until I discovered the true impact of oxalates on health that everything began to make sense. I started eliminating high-oxalate foods from my diet, and the changes were nothing short of miraculous. My energy returned, the pain subsided, and for the first time in years, I felt like myself again. This journey opened my eyes to a simple but groundbreaking truth: what we've been told about "healthy" eating isn't always the whole story.

If you're dealing with unexplained fatigue, pain, inflammation, or even mental health struggles like anxiety and brain fog, the answer might not lie in doing more of what you've been taught. It could be in removing what you thought was good for you. This book, The Toxic Superfoods Cookbook, is here to help you do just that.

Inside, you'll discover:

The surprising truth about oxalates lurking in popular superfoods

How these toxins could be the root cause of your chronic health issues

A safe, science-backed plan to detox your body from oxalates

Delicious, low-oxalate recipes that nourish and heal without compromising flavour or enjoyment

Whether you've been trying to manage chronic pain, improve your mental clarity, or simply feel more energetic, this book provides the missing piece of the puzzle. Through research-backed information and practical, easy-to-follow recipes, you'll learn how to reclaim your health—and thrive in ways you never thought possible.

Your path to relief, energy, and vitality starts here. It's time to stop poisoning yourself with the wrong "superfoods" and start eating the right way for your body. Ready to make the change? Let's begin.

Understanding Toxic Superfoods

In today's health-conscious world, we are constantly bombarded with messages about the benefits of eating more plants. From leafy greens to nuts and seeds, the idea is that the more plant-based foods we consume, the healthier we will be. Superfoods like spinach, almonds, sweet potatoes, and chia seeds have earned their place in health circles as nutrient-dense foods, rich in vitamins, minerals, and antioxidants. We're told that eating these foods will reduce our risk of chronic diseases, boost our energy levels, and help us live longer, healthier lives.

But what if these superfoods aren't as super as we've been led to believe?

The truth is, some of the most highly regarded "health foods" could be contributing to your fatigue, inflammation, and chronic pain. Beneath their glowing reputations, certain plant foods contain naturally occurring compounds that can be harmful when consumed in large amounts. One of the most notorious of these compounds is oxalate, a toxic chemical that accumulates in your body over time, potentially leading to an array of health problems.

Oxalates are present in many of the most popular superfoods. While it's true that these foods contain beneficial nutrients, they also carry a hidden risk: oxalates can bind with minerals like calcium and magnesium, creating crystals that lodge in various tissues throughout the body. These crystals can cause damage to the kidneys, bones, joints, and even the brain. If you've been eating a so-called healthy diet and still find yourself struggling with unexplained health issues, oxalates could be the culprit.

In this section of the book, we'll dive deep into what makes these seemingly healthy foods toxic for some people. We'll explore why oxalates have been overlooked in the conversation about nutrition, and how they can quietly contribute to everything from kidney stones to arthritis to chronic fatigue. By understanding the hidden dangers of toxic superfoods, you'll be better equipped to make informed decisions about what you put on your plate and how you can protect your health moving forward.

My Journey to Wellness: From Superfoods to Healing

For years, I followed every bit of conventional wisdom when it came to eating healthy. I filled my diet with vibrant salads, green smoothies, and nutrient-rich snacks like almonds and sweet potatoes. I avoided processed foods, limited my sugar intake, and stuck to what I believed was a clean, plant-based way of eating. On paper, I was doing everything right. But in reality, my body was in turmoil.

It started gradually—mild fatigue, digestive discomfort, the occasional headache. Over time, the symptoms worsened. I felt perpetually exhausted, even though I was eating foods designed to boost energy. My joints ached, my muscles were sore, and I started experiencing sharp, inexplicable pains in different parts of my body. Doctors prescribed medications for inflammation and pain, but nothing seemed to address the root cause. Worst of all, I developed kidney stones, which only added to the stress and confusion.

I couldn't understand it. I was eating a "perfect" diet—why was my body breaking down?

Desperate for answers, I began researching my symptoms and stumbled upon a revelation that would change my life: oxalates. I learned that these compounds, found in many of the foods I was eating in large quantities, could accumulate in the body and lead to chronic health issues. Oxalates are found in foods like spinach, almonds, beets, sweet potatoes, and dark chocolate—all of which I consumed regularly, believing they were doing me good.

I decided to make a radical change. I eliminated high-oxalate foods from my diet and introduced low-oxalate alternatives. Within weeks, the fog began to lift. My energy returned, the chronic pain subsided, and my digestive issues started to resolve. Over time, my health improved in ways I hadn't imagined possible. The key had been there all along—hiding in the foods I thought were healing me.

This personal journey opened my eyes to the dangers of oxalates, and it became my mission to share this knowledge with others. I wasn't alone. There were countless others suffering in silence, struggling with unexplained symptoms, who had no idea that their "healthy" diet could be the source of their pain. That's why I created this book—to guide you through the process of identifying toxic superfoods in your diet and provide the tools you need to reclaim your health, just as I did.

What Are Oxalates?

Oxalates, or oxalic acid, are naturally occurring compounds found in many plant foods. While they serve a useful function in plants, primarily as a defence mechanism against herbivores, oxalates can have damaging effects on the human body. In small amounts, oxalates are usually harmless and are excreted in the urine without causing harm. However, when consumed in large amounts, or if your body has difficulty eliminating them, oxalates can accumulate and lead to serious health problems.

Oxalates are known for their ability to bind with minerals like calcium, forming sharp, needle-like crystals. These crystals can lodge in various tissues, including the kidneys, joints, and even the skin, causing irritation, inflammation, and pain. One of the most common health issues associated with oxalates is kidney stones, which are often composed of calcium oxalate crystals.

However, kidney stones are just the tip of the iceberg. Oxalates have also been linked to:

- Joint pain and arthritis-like symptoms
- Muscle weakness and fatigue
- Digestive issues, including bloating, gas, and discomfort
- Brain fog, anxiety, and mood disorders
- Bone thinning and osteoporosis
- Skin rashes and irritation

The effects of oxalates can vary depending on individual sensitivity. Some people can eat high-oxalate foods with no apparent issues, while others may experience significant health challenges even with moderate consumption. Genetics, gut health, and the ability of the body to detoxify oxalates all play a role in determining how oxalates affect you.

Unfortunately, many of the foods that are highest in oxalates are also considered superfoods—spinach, almonds, beets, sweet potatoes, and even turmeric contain significant levels of oxalates. This means that people who are trying to eat a clean, plant-based diet may inadvertently be consuming large amounts of oxalates on a daily basis, setting themselves up for chronic health issues.

The good news is that by understanding where oxalates come from and how they affect the body, you can make informed choices about the foods you eat and take steps to reduce your oxalate load.

The Modern Diet: A Plant-Based Paradox

In recent years, plant-based diets have become the gold standard for health. We're told to eat more plants, avoid animal products, and focus on consuming nutrient-dense foods like vegetables, legumes, nuts, and seeds. While there's no denying that plants provide essential vitamins, minerals, and antioxidants, there's a dark side to this trend that many people don't realise: the rise of oxalates.

As more people shift towards plant-based eating, they are unknowingly increasing their intake of oxalates, which can accumulate in the body and cause damage over time. The paradox is clear: the very foods we've been told will enhance our health may actually be undermining it.

Spinach is often celebrated for its high levels of iron and calcium, but it also contains one of the highest concentrations of oxalates of any food. Almonds, a favourite snack for those avoiding dairy, are also packed with oxalates. Sweet potatoes, touted as a nutrient-rich alternative to white potatoes, are another common source of oxalates. Even green smoothies, the poster child for clean eating, can be a major oxalate trap when they include ingredients like spinach, beets, and kale.

The problem isn't just that these foods contain oxalates—it's that modern eating patterns encourage overconsumption of them. Smoothies and salads, once a day or more, can lead to a dangerous oxalate buildup. Combine this with the widespread use of almond-based products (almond milk, almond flour, almond butter), and it's easy to see how a well-intentioned diet can turn into a health disaster.

The rise of plant-based diets also coincides with an increase in certain health problems—kidney stones, joint pain, chronic inflammation, and digestive disorders—all of which are linked to oxalate toxicity. Could it be that our shift towards eating more plants has unintentionally worsened our health?

This is not to say that plant-based diets are inherently harmful, but it is crucial to understand that not all plants are created equal. By learning to identify high-oxalate foods and replacing them with low-oxalate alternatives, you can enjoy the benefits of a nutrient-rich diet without the negative effects of oxalates.

The goal of this book is to help you navigate the modern diet paradox and make informed decisions about the foods you eat. You don't have to give up on eating plants—just the ones that are hurting you.

Chapter 1: The Science Behind Oxalates and Your Health

The narrative surrounding health foods often emphasises the importance of incorporating more plant-based foods into our diets for optimal well-being. Leafy greens, nuts, seeds, and root vegetables have long been lauded as "superfoods," praised for their nutrient density and the array of vitamins, minerals, and antioxidants they provide. Yet, beneath the surface, many of these celebrated foods harbour a hidden risk: oxalates.

Oxalates are naturally occurring compounds found in many plants that serve as a defence mechanism against herbivores. While they protect the plants, they can also pose significant health risks to humans, especially when consumed in large amounts. This chapter will explore the science behind oxalates, shedding light on how these compounds can disrupt your health, affect the gut, impact brain function, and why genetics and individual sensitivity play a crucial role in how oxalates affect each person.

The Link Between Oxalates and Chronic Disease

Chronic diseases such as kidney stones, arthritis, and even autoimmune disorders have been linked to oxalate toxicity. One of the most well-known issues related to oxalates is their role in kidney stones. Oxalates bind with calcium in the body to form insoluble calcium oxalate crystals, which are responsible for 80% of all kidney stones. The accumulation of these crystals can lead to pain, discomfort, and serious kidney damage.

But kidney stones are just the beginning. Research indicates that oxalates may contribute to a variety of chronic conditions by creating inflammation and oxidative stress in the body. Here are some of the most significant health concerns linked to oxalate toxicity:

Inflammation and Joint Pain: Oxalates are known to deposit in tissues, including joints and muscles, potentially leading to inflammation and pain. Many people suffering from conditions like arthritis or fibromyalgia report improvements after reducing their intake of high-oxalate foods.

Autoimmune Disorders: The link between oxalates and autoimmune diseases is becoming clearer as more research emerges. Oxalates can provoke the immune system, causing a heightened inflammatory response, which may trigger or worsen autoimmune conditions like lupus, rheumatoid arthritis, and celiac disease.

Kidney Health: Beyond kidney stones, oxalates can lead to broader kidney dysfunction by damaging delicate kidney tissues. This can impair the body's ability to filter waste, leading to further toxic buildup.

Chronic Fatigue and Fibromyalgia: Many individuals with chronic fatigue syndrome (CFS) or fibromyalgia have discovered that high levels of oxalates in their diets were contributing to their symptoms. The accumulation of oxalates in muscles and connective tissue can cause significant pain and fatigue.

The body has mechanisms in place to excrete oxalates through urine and stool, but when the system is overloaded, or the body's ability to detoxify oxalates is compromised, these toxins begin to build up in tissues, causing chronic disease over time. The damage caused by oxalates often goes unnoticed for years, leading to a gradual worsening of symptoms that are difficult to diagnose.

How Oxalates Disrupt Gut Health

The gut is often called the "second brain" of the body, and for good reason—it's where digestion occurs, nutrients are absorbed, and a significant portion of the immune system is located. However, oxalates can wreak havoc on gut health by disrupting digestion, damaging the intestinal lining, and interfering with nutrient absorption.

Here's how oxalates negatively affect gut health:

Leaky Gut Syndrome: Oxalates can irritate the intestinal lining, leading to increased intestinal permeability, also known as "leaky gut." When this happens, toxins, undigested food particles, and harmful bacteria can pass through the gut barrier and enter the bloodstream, triggering systemic inflammation and immune responses.

Nutrient Malabsorption: Oxalates bind with minerals such as calcium, magnesium, and iron, preventing their absorption in the intestines. Over time, this can lead to mineral deficiencies that contribute to a wide range of health problems, including weak bones, fatigue, and impaired immune function.

Disruption of Gut Microbiome: The gut microbiome, composed of trillions of beneficial bacteria, plays a crucial role in maintaining overall health. Unfortunately, high levels of oxalates can disrupt the balance of these bacteria, leading to dysbiosis (an imbalance in gut flora) and an increased risk of digestive issues such as bloating, gas, constipation, and diarrhoea.

Exacerbation of Digestive Disorders: For individuals with pre-existing digestive conditions, such as irritable bowel syndrome (IBS), Crohn's disease, or celiac disease, high-oxalate foods can worsen symptoms by further irritating the already compromised digestive tract.

In addition to these direct impacts, oxalates can contribute to the development of food intolerances and sensitivities by inflaming the gut and weakening the body's ability to process certain foods. Over time, this can create a vicious cycle, where the body reacts negatively to an increasing number of foods, further compromising health.

Oxalates and Brain Health: Impact on Mood and Cognitive Function

The connection between oxalates and brain health is an emerging area of research, but the evidence so far suggests that oxalates can have a significant impact on mood, cognitive function, and mental clarity. The brain is highly sensitive to inflammation and oxidative stress, and oxalates can exacerbate both of these issues.

Here are some of the key ways oxalates affect brain health:

Mood Disorders: Oxalates have been linked to mood imbalances such as anxiety, depression, and irritability. The inflammation caused by oxalates can interfere with neurotransmitter production and function, particularly serotonin, which is critical for regulating mood and promoting a sense of well-being.

Brain Fog: Many people who struggle with oxalate toxicity report experiencing brain fog, characterised by difficulty concentrating, memory problems, and a general sense of mental fatigue. This cognitive impairment is likely due to the oxidative stress that oxalates place on the brain.

Neurological Symptoms: In severe cases, oxalate buildup in the nervous system can lead to neurological symptoms such as tingling, numbness, and even neuropathy. This occurs when oxalates form crystals in nerve tissues, causing damage to the nerves and impairing their function.

Impaired Detoxification: The brain relies on the body's detoxification pathways to remove harmful substances. When oxalates overload the system, it can slow down detoxification processes, allowing other toxins to accumulate in the brain, further contributing to cognitive and mood-related issues.

The gut-brain axis plays a crucial role in mood regulation and cognitive function. As previously mentioned, oxalates can disrupt gut health, leading to a cascade of effects on the brain. This explains why individuals with high oxalate loads often experience both digestive problems and mental health challenges. By addressing oxalate toxicity, it's possible to not only improve physical health but also enhance mental clarity, focus, and emotional well-being.

Understanding the Role of Genetics and Individual Sensitivity

While oxalates can affect anyone, individual sensitivity to oxalates varies greatly. Some people can consume high-oxalate foods without experiencing noticeable symptoms, while others may suffer from severe reactions after consuming even small amounts of oxalates. This variation is largely due to genetics and the body's ability to process and eliminate oxalates.

Here are some of the factors that influence how oxalates affect individuals:

Genetic Variations: Certain genetic factors can make individuals more prone to oxalate accumulation. For example, mutations in genes responsible for oxalate metabolism or detoxification may lead to a reduced ability to break down and eliminate oxalates from the body. This can result in a higher risk of developing oxalate-related health issues such as kidney stones or joint pain.

Gut Health: The health of the gut microbiome plays a critical role in determining how well the body can handle oxalates. Some beneficial bacteria, such as Oxalobacter formigenes, have the ability to break down oxalates in the intestines before they can be absorbed into the bloodstream. However, the use of antibiotics, a poor diet, or gut dysbiosis can reduce the population of these bacteria, making individuals more susceptible to oxalate toxicity.

Detoxification Pathways: The body's ability to detoxify and eliminate oxalates varies from person to person. Factors such as liver function, kidney health, and hydration levels all play a role in determining how efficiently oxalates are excreted. For individuals with compromised detoxification pathways, oxalates can accumulate more quickly, leading to an increased risk of chronic health issues.

Oxalate Sensitivity: Just as some people are more sensitive to gluten or lactose, others may be more sensitive to oxalates. Oxalate sensitivity can manifest in a wide range of symptoms, from digestive discomfort and joint pain to headaches and fatigue. For these individuals, even small amounts of oxalates can trigger significant health problems.

Understanding your personal sensitivity to oxalates is key to managing your health. For some, it may be necessary to adopt a low-oxalate diet to prevent oxalate buildup and reduce the risk of chronic disease. For others, simply reducing the intake of high-oxalate foods or supporting gut health may be enough to mitigate the effects of oxalates.

In conclusion, oxalates are a hidden threat lurking in many of the foods we've been taught to view as healthy. By understanding the science behind oxalates and how they affect the body, you can make informed decisions about your diet and take steps to protect your health. Whether you're struggling with chronic disease, digestive issues, or brain fog, addressing oxalate toxicity may be the missing piece of the puzzle in your journey to optimal well-being.

Chapter 2: Detoxing from Oxalates – A Step-by-Step Guide

Detoxing from oxalates is not a simple "cold turkey" process. Unlike other dietary changes, the transition to a low-oxalate diet requires careful planning, gradual shifts, and an understanding of how your body will react. Oxalates have a way of accumulating in the body, especially in tissues like the kidneys, bones, muscles, and even the brain. Therefore, reducing oxalate intake too quickly can lead to unpleasant withdrawal symptoms as stored oxalates are released back into the bloodstream.

In this chapter, we will walk you through the process of transitioning to a low-oxalate diet, outline what to expect during this change, discuss how to safely lower your oxalate load, and provide practical healing strategies to support your body during oxalate detox.

Transitioning to a Low-Oxalate Diet: What to Expect

When transitioning to a low-oxalate diet, it's essential to approach the change slowly and carefully. Oxalates are stored in the body over time, so if you drastically cut high-oxalate foods from your diet, the body can begin to release these stored oxalates too quickly. This can lead to a temporary worsening of symptoms, known as "oxalate dumping," which occurs when oxalates are flushed out of tissues and into circulation for elimination.

Here's what to expect as you begin transitioning:

Gradual Reduction Is Key: Cutting oxalates from your diet too abruptly can cause a sudden release of stored oxalates into the bloodstream, leading to unpleasant side effects.

The safest approach is to gradually reduce your oxalate intake over weeks or even months. Aim to decrease oxalates by 5-10% per week until you reach your target.

Oxalate Dumping: As you lower your oxalate intake, your body will begin to release oxalates that have accumulated in tissues. This release can lead to a temporary increase in symptoms, such as fatigue, joint pain, digestive discomfort, and skin rashes. It's important to recognize that these symptoms are a sign that your body is detoxing and adjusting.

Energy Fluctuations: During the initial stages of oxalate detox, some people report feeling more fatigued or experiencing brain fog. This is often due to the body adapting to lower oxalate levels and processing the release of stored oxalates.

Improved Symptoms Over Time: While the initial phase of detoxing from oxalates can be challenging, most people begin to notice improvements in their symptoms after a few weeks or months. Joint pain, fatigue, digestive problems, and other issues associated with oxalate toxicity often lessen or disappear altogether as the body eliminates oxalates more effectively.

As you move forward with reducing oxalates in your diet, it's important to listen to your body. If symptoms become overwhelming, you may need to slow down the pace of your detox. Every person's tolerance to oxalate detox is different, so pay attention to how you feel and adjust your plan accordingly.

How to Safely Lower Your Oxalate Load

When it comes to safely lowering your oxalate load, a strategic approach is essential. Because high-oxalate foods can be found in so many plant-based staples, such as spinach, sweet potatoes, almonds, and chocolate, it can feel overwhelming to figure out where to start. The following steps provide a roadmap for gradually lowering your oxalate load while minimising potential side effects.

Identify High-Oxalate Foods: The first step in lowering your oxalate load is to become familiar with high-oxalate foods. Common culprits include spinach, beets, sweet potatoes, nuts (especially almonds and cashews), seeds, rhubarb, buckwheat, quinoa, and certain fruits like kiwi and raspberries. Start by identifying the high-oxalate foods in your current diet and creating a plan to reduce them gradually.

Transition Slowly: Once you've identified the foods that contribute to a high oxalate load, begin reducing them slowly. For example, if you're eating spinach salads daily, swap out spinach for lower-oxalate greens like arugula, romaine, or iceberg lettuce. If you regularly snack on almonds, try switching to low-oxalate nuts like macadamias or pecans. Reducing high-oxalate foods step by step will help your body adjust without overwhelming it.

Stay Hydrated: Drinking plenty of water is critical when detoxing from oxalates. Proper hydration helps your kidneys flush oxalates from the body, reducing the likelihood of oxalate crystal formation and promoting detoxification. Aim for at least 8-10 cups of water per day, and consider incorporating hydrating herbal teas like chamomile or peppermint.

Balance Calcium Intake: Calcium binds with oxalates in the digestive tract, preventing them from being absorbed into the bloodstream. To help lower your oxalate load, ensure you're getting enough calcium from your diet, preferably from low-oxalate sources. Good options include dairy products like yogurt and cheese, as well as calcium-rich vegetables like broccoli and kale.

Incorporate Citrate: Citrate, found in foods like lemons and limes, can inhibit the formation of calcium oxalate crystals. Squeezing lemon or lime juice over salads, in water, or in cooking can help reduce oxalate absorption and support your detox efforts.

Include Probiotic-Rich Foods: The gut microbiome plays a crucial role in oxalate detoxification, as certain beneficial bacteria help break down oxalates in the intestines. Including fermented foods like yoghourt, kefir, sauerkraut, and kimchi can promote a healthy gut environment and support the body's ability to eliminate oxalates.

Monitor Symptoms and Adjust: As you lower your oxalate intake, it's essential to monitor how your body responds. If you experience severe detox symptoms, slow down the pace of your transition. On the other hand, if your symptoms improve, you may feel comfortable reducing oxalates more quickly. Keeping a food and symptom journal can help you track your progress and identify which changes are most beneficial for you.

Oxalate Detox Symptoms: What You Need to Know

Detoxing from oxalates can come with a range of symptoms that vary in intensity from person to person. These symptoms, often referred to as "oxalate dumping," occur when stored oxalates are released from tissues and enter the bloodstream for elimination. While uncomfortable, these symptoms are a natural part of the detox process and typically subside over time as the body adjusts.

Here are some common oxalate detox symptoms to be aware of:

Joint and Muscle Pain: As oxalates leave tissues where they've been stored, they can cause temporary joint and muscle pain. This is especially common in individuals with a history of arthritis, fibromyalgia, or other musculoskeletal issues. The pain can range from mild to severe and may move around the body.

Digestive Distress: Oxalate detox can affect the digestive system, leading to symptoms such as bloating, gas, diarrhoea, or constipation. Some individuals also report experiencing nausea or cramping as their bodies adjust to lower oxalate levels.

Skin Issues: Oxalate crystals can be expelled through the skin, leading to rashes, itching, or even small bumps that resemble pimples. These skin issues are typically short-lived and clear up once the body has flushed out excess oxalates.

Fatigue and Brain Fog: During the detox process, some individuals experience fatigue, brain fog, or difficulty concentrating. These symptoms are often linked to the body's efforts to process and eliminate oxalates, as well as the temporary imbalance caused by the release of stored toxins.

Flare-Ups of Pre-Existing Conditions: For those with chronic health conditions, oxalate detox can sometimes trigger a temporary worsening of symptoms. This is especially common in individuals with autoimmune diseases, digestive disorders, or inflammatory conditions.

Increased Urination: As oxalates are processed by the kidneys, many people notice an increase in urination frequency or changes in urine color. Drinking plenty of water can help support the kidneys during this detox phase.

While these symptoms can be uncomfortable, they are usually temporary and can be managed with supportive strategies, which we'll explore in the next section. It's important to remember that detox symptoms are a sign that your body is healing and adjusting to lower oxalate levels.

Healing Strategies: Supporting Your Body Through Oxalate Withdrawal

Detoxing from oxalates can be challenging, but with the right strategies, you can support your body and minimise the discomfort associated with oxalate withdrawal. The key to a successful detox lies in providing your body with the nutrients, hydration, and support it needs to efficiently eliminate oxalates and heal from their toxic effects.

Here are some effective healing strategies to help you navigate the detox process:

Stay Hydrated: As mentioned earlier, drinking plenty of water is crucial for flushing oxalates from your system. In addition to water, you can include herbal teas like nettle, dandelion, or chamomile, which have gentle detoxifying properties and support kidney function.

Support Your Kidneys: The kidneys play a vital role in oxalate elimination. To support kidney health during detox, consider incorporating foods and supplements that promote kidney function. Herbal teas such as marshmallow root, dandelion, and uva ursi are known for their kidney-supporting properties. Adequate magnesium intake is also important, as magnesium can help prevent the formation of oxalate crystals.

Optimise Gut Health: Since the gut plays a key role in oxalate detox, it's important to prioritise gut health during this process. Probiotic-rich foods like yoghourt, kefir, sauerkraut, and kimchi can help maintain a healthy balance of gut bacteria that aid in oxalate breakdown.

You can also consider taking a probiotic supplement with strains like Lactobacillus and Bifidobacterium, which have been shown to support oxalate metabolism.

Balance Electrolytes: Detoxing from oxalates can sometimes lead to an imbalance in electrolytes, especially if you experience increased urination or digestive upset. To restore electrolyte balance, focus on consuming potassium-rich foods like bananas, avocados, and leafy greens, as well as magnesium-rich foods such as nuts, seeds, and whole grains.

Eat a Nutrient-Dense Diet: While you're detoxing from oxalates, it's important to nourish your body with a nutrient-dense, anti-inflammatory diet. Focus on whole, unprocessed foods that are low in oxalates, such as lean proteins, non-starchy vegetables, healthy fats, and low-oxalate fruits like berries and citrus. These foods will provide the vitamins, minerals, and antioxidants your body needs to repair and regenerate.

Rest and Relaxation: Detoxing can be physically and emotionally taxing, so it's important to give your body plenty of rest. Ensure you're getting adequate sleep each night, and incorporate relaxation techniques like deep breathing, meditation, or gentle yoga to help reduce stress and support healing.

Magnesium and Calcium Supplements: As magnesium and calcium are known to help bind oxalates in the digestive tract and prevent their absorption, consider taking supplements under the guidance of a healthcare provider. Magnesium citrate and calcium citrate are two forms that are particularly effective in reducing oxalate levels.

Manage Detox Symptoms with Epsom Salt Baths: Taking regular Epsom salt baths can help ease muscle aches, joint pain, and fatigue associated with oxalate detox. The magnesium sulphate in Epsom salt is absorbed through the skin and can help relax muscles, reduce inflammation, and promote detoxification.

By incorporating these healing strategies into your detox routine, you can support your body through the process of eliminating oxalates and reduce the severity of withdrawal symptoms. Remember, detoxing from oxalates is a gradual process, and it's important to give your body the time it needs to heal.

Chapter 3: Low-Oxalate Breakfasts to Heal and Thrive

Scrambled Eggs with Mushrooms and Spinach

Servings: 1

Ingredients:

2 large eggs

1/2 cup mushrooms, chopped

1/4 cup baby spinach

1 tbsp olive oil

Salt and pepper to taste

Preparation:

Get olive oil heated in a pan over medium heat.

Have the mushrooms added and cook until soft (about 3-4 minutes).

Add spinach and cook until wilted.

In a separate bowl, whisk eggs, then pour into the pan with veggies.

Stir gently until eggs are scrambled and fully cooked. Season with salt and pepper.

Nutritional Information (per serving):

Calories: 230 kcal

Protein: 13 g

Fat: 18 g

Carbohydrates: 3 g

Fibre: 1 g

Oxalates: 5 mg

Coconut Chia Pudding

Servings: 1

Ingredients:

1/4 cup chia seeds

3/4 cup coconut milk

1 tsp vanilla extract

1/2 tsp cinnamon

1 tbsp maple syrup

Preparation:

Mix chia seeds, coconut milk, vanilla, cinnamon, and maple syrup in a bowl.

Stir well and let sit for 5 minutes. Stir again to prevent clumping.

Cover and refrigerate overnight.

Serve cold, topped with low-oxalate fruits like strawberries.

Nutritional Information (per serving):

Calories: 310 kcal

Protein: 5 g

Fat: 22 g

Carbohydrates: 24 g

Fibre: 9 g

Oxalates: 8 mg

Almond Butter Oatmeal

Servings: 1

Ingredients:

1/2 cup gluten-free oats

1 cup water or milk (dairy or almond)

1 tbsp almond butter

1/2 tsp cinnamon

1 tsp honey

1/4 tsp vanilla extract

Preparation:

In a pot, bring water or milk to a boil, then add oats.

Lower heat and simmer until oats are cooked (about 5 minutes).

Stir in almond butter, cinnamon, honey, and vanilla. Mix until creamy.

Serve warm.

Nutritional Information (per serving):

Calories: 320 kcal

Protein: 8 g

Fat: 14 g

Carbohydrates: 39 g

Fibre: 5 g

Oxalates: 10 mg

Greek Yoghourt with Blueberries and Honey

Servings: 1

Ingredients:

1 cup plain Greek yoghourt

1/4 cup blueberries

1 tsp honey

1 tbsp flaxseeds

Preparation:

Scoop Greek yogurt into a bowl.

Top with fresh blueberries, drizzle with honey, and sprinkle flaxseeds on top.

Serve chilled.

Nutritional Information (per serving):

Calories: 230 kcal

Protein: 16 g

Fat: 8 g

Carbohydrates: 22 g

Fibre: 3 g

Oxalates: 5 mg

Zucchini Egg Muffins

Servings: 6 muffins

Ingredients:

4 large eggs

1/2 cup zucchini, grated

1/4 cup cheddar cheese, shredded

1/4 tsp garlic powder

Salt and pepper to taste

Preparation:

Preheat oven to 350°F (175°C) and have a muffin tin greased.

In a bowl, whisk eggs, then add zucchini, cheese, garlic powder, salt, and pepper.

Pour mixture into muffin tin, filling each cup halfway.

Bake for 15-20 minutes until muffins are set and lightly browned.

Let it cool, then remove from the tin.

Nutritional Information (per muffin):

Calories: 80 kcal

Protein: 6 g

Fat: 5 g

Carbohydrates: 2 g

Fibre: 0.5 g

Oxalates: 3 mg

Coconut Flour Pancakes

Servings: 1

Ingredients:

2 tbsp coconut flour

2 large eggs

1/4 cup almond milk

1/2 tsp baking powder

1/4 tsp vanilla extract

1 tbsp coconut oil for frying

Preparation:

In a bowl, mix eggs, almond milk, and vanilla extract.

Stir in coconut flour and baking powder until smooth.

Heat coconut oil in a skillet and pour in pancake batter, cooking each side for 2-3 minutes until golden brown.

Serve with butter or low-oxalate fruits like berries.

Nutritional Information (per serving):

Calories: 280 kcal

Protein: 11 g

Fat: 22 g

Carbohydrates: 9 g

Fibre: 5 g

Oxalates: 6 mg

Avocado and Poached Egg Toast

Servings: 1

Ingredients:

1 slice sourdough bread

1/2 avocado

1 poached egg

Salt, pepper, and red pepper flakes to taste

Preparation:

Toast the sourdough bread.

Get the avocado mashed and spread it on the toast.

Top with a poached egg and spice using salt, pepper, and red pepper flakes.

Serve immediately.

Nutritional Information (per serving):

Calories: 350 kcal

Protein: 10 g

Fat: 24 g

Carbohydrates: 26 g

Fibre: 6 g

Oxalates: 5 mg

Low-Oxalate Green Smoothie

Servings: 1

Ingredients:

1/2 cup cucumber

1/2 cup kale

1/2 green apple

1/2 cup coconut water

1 tbsp chia seeds

Preparation:

Get all the ingredients combined in a blender and blend until smooth.
Serve chilled.

Nutritional Information (per serving):

Calories: 150 kcal

Protein: 3 g

Fat: 4 g

Carbohydrates: 30 g

Fibre: 6 g

Oxalates: 8 mg

Sweet Potato Hash with Turkey Sausage

Servings: 2

Ingredients:

1 cup diced sweet potatoes

1 turkey sausage, sliced

1/2 bell pepper, diced

1/4 onion, diced

1 tbsp olive oil

Salt and pepper to taste

Preparation:

Get the olive oil heated in a skillet over medium heat.

Add sweet potatoes, cooking until softened.

Add sausage, bell pepper, and onion. Cook until browned and cooked through.

Season with salt and pepper.

Nutritional Information (per serving):

Calories: 260 kcal

Protein: 12 g

Fat: 10 g

Carbohydrates: 30 g

Fibre: 4 g

Oxalates: 12 mg

Berry Yogurt Smoothie

Servings: 1

Ingredients:

1/2 cup plain Greek yogurt

1/4 cup strawberries

1/4 cup blueberries

1/2 cup almond milk

1 tsp honey

Preparation:

Blend all ingredients together until smooth.

Serve chilled.

Nutritional Information (per serving):

Calories: 180 kcal

Protein: 9 g

Fat: 5 g

Carbohydrates: 27 g

Fibre: 3 g

Oxalates: 8 mg

Cottage Cheese and Pineapple Bowl

Servings: 1

Ingredients:

1/2 cup cottage cheese

1/4 cup diced pineapple

1 tsp chia seeds

Preparation:

In a bowl, combine cottage cheese, pineapple, and chia seeds.
Serve chilled.

Nutritional Information (per serving):

Calories: 140 kcal

Protein: 11 g

Fat: 3 g

Carbohydrates: 16 g

Fibre: 2 g

Oxalates: 5 mg

Egg and Bacon Breakfast Wrap

Servings: 1

Ingredients:

1 large egg

1 slice turkey bacon

1 low-carb tortilla

1 tbsp salsa

Preparation:

Cook egg and bacon in a skillet.

Place cooked egg and bacon inside the tortilla.

Add salsa, wrap, and serve.

Nutritional Information (per serving):

Calories: 220 kcal

Protein: 12 g

Fat: 12 g

Carbohydrates: 18 g

Fibre: 3 g

Oxalates: 4 mg

Pumpkin Seed Porridge

Servings: 1

Ingredients:

1/4 cup pumpkin seeds

1/2 cup almond milk

1 tbsp chia seeds

1 tsp cinnamon

Preparation:

Blend pumpkin seeds until fine, then mix with almond milk, chia seeds, and cinnamon.

Heat on the stovetop until thickened.

Serve warm.

Nutritional Information (per serving):

Calories: 190 kcal

Protein: 7 g

Fat: 12 g

Carbohydrates: 15 g

Fibre: 5 g

Oxalates: 7 mg

Cucumber and Smoked Salmon Bagel

Servings: 1

Ingredients:

1 whole wheat bagel

2 oz smoked salmon

1/4 cucumber, sliced

1 tbsp cream cheese

Preparation:

Get the bagel toasted and spread with cream cheese.

Layer smoked salmon and cucumber on top.

Serve immediately.

Nutritional Information (per serving):

Calories: 350 kcal

Protein: 16 g

Fat: 12 g

Carbohydrates: 42 g

Fibre: 4 g

Oxalates: 6 mg

Flaxseed Porridge

Servings: 1

Ingredients:

2 tbsp ground flaxseed

1/2 cup coconut milk

1 tsp vanilla extract

1 tbsp almond butter

1 tsp cinnamon

Preparation:

In a saucepan, heat coconut milk and stir in flaxseed, vanilla, and cinnamon.

Simmer for 3-4 minutes until thickened.

Top with almond butter and serve.

Nutritional Information (per serving):

Calories: 250 kcal

Protein: 7 g

Fat: 19 g

Carbohydrates: 13 g

Fibre: 7 g

Oxalates. 9 mg

Chapter 4: Oxalate-Free Lunches

Grilled Chicken Salad

Servings: 2

Ingredients:

2 grilled chicken breasts (6 oz each)

4 cups romaine lettuce, chopped

1/2 cucumber, sliced

1/4 cup bell peppers, chopped

1/4 cup feta cheese, crumbled

2 tbsp olive oil

1 tbsp lemon juice

Salt and pepper to taste

Preparation:

Grill chicken breasts until cooked through and slice them.

In a large bowl, combine lettuce, cucumber, bell peppers, and feta.

Drizzle with olive oil and lemon juice. Toss to combine.

Top with sliced chicken, season with salt and pepper, and serve.

Nutritional Information (per serving):

Calories: 450 kcal

Protein: 40 g

Fat: 30 g

Carbohydrates: 10 g

Fibre: 2 g

Oxalates: 0 mg

Turkey and Cheese Roll-Ups

Servings: 2

Ingredients:

4 slices turkey breast

4 slices cheddar cheese

1/2 avocado, sliced

1/4 cup bell pepper, sliced

1 tbsp mayonnaise

Preparation:

Lay out turkey slices and place a slice of cheese on each.

Top with avocado and bell pepper slices.

Spread mayonnaise, roll them up, and secure with toothpicks if desired.

Nutritional Information (per serving):

Calories: 300 kcal

Protein: 30 g

Fat: 18 g

Carbohydrates: 8 g

Fibre: 3 g

Oxalates: 0 mg

Quinoa and Vegetable Stir-Fry

Servings: 2

Ingredients:

1 cup cooked quinoa

1 cup broccoli florets

1/2 cup bell peppers, chopped

1/2 cup carrots, sliced

2 tbsp olive oil

1 tbsp soy sauce (gluten-free)

Salt and pepper to taste

Preparation:

Get the olive oil heated in a skillet over medium heat.

Add broccoli, bell peppers, and carrots. Sauté for 5-7 minutes until tender.

Stir in cooked quinoa and soy sauce, cooking until heated through.

Season with salt and pepper before serving.

Nutritional Information (per serving):

Calories: 350 kcal

Protein: 10 g

Fat: 14 g

Carbohydrates: 50 g

Fibre: 6 g

Oxalates: 0 mg

Egg Salad Lettuce Wraps

Servings: 2

Ingredients:

4 large eggs, hard-boiled and chopped

2 tbsp mayonnaise

1 tsp mustard

1/4 cup celery, diced

Salt and pepper to taste

8 large lettuce leaves

Preparation:

In a bowl, mix chopped eggs, mayonnaise, mustard, celery, salt, and pepper until combined.

Get the egg salad spooned into lettuce leaves and wrap them.

Serve immediately.

Nutritional Information (per serving):

Calories: 250 kcal

Protein: 18 g

Fat: 18 g

Carbohydrates: 2 g

Fibre: 1 g

Oxalates: 0 mg

Zucchini Noodles with Marinara Sauce

Servings: 2

Ingredients:

2 medium zucchinis, spiralized

1 cup marinara sauce (store-bought, low-sugar)

1/4 cup parmesan cheese, grated

1 tbsp olive oil

Salt and pepper to taste

Preparation:

Get the olive oil heated in a skillet over medium heat. Get the zucchini noodles added and cook for 3-4 minutes until slightly softened.

Add marinara sauce, stirring to combine, and cook until heated through.

Top using the grated parmesan cheese and season with salt and pepper, and enjoy.

Nutritional Information (per serving):

Calories: 220 kcal

Protein: 8 g

Fat: 14 g

Carbohydrates: 20 g

Fibre: 4 g

Oxalates: 2 mg

Shrimp and Asparagus Stir-Fry

Servings: 2

Ingredients:

8 oz shrimp, peeled and deveined

1 cup asparagus, chopped

1/2 cup bell peppers, sliced

2 tbsp olive oil

2 cloves garlic, minced

Salt and pepper to taste

Preparation:

Get the olive oil heated in a skillet over medium heat. Add garlic and cook until fragrant.

Get the shrimp added and cook until pink (about 2-3 minutes).

Add asparagus and bell peppers, cooking until tender.

Season with salt and pepper before serving.

Nutritional Information (per serving):

Calories: 300 kcal

Protein: 30 g

Fat: 18 g

Carbohydrates: 10 g

Fibre: 3 g

Oxalates: 0 mg

Cauliflower Rice Bowl

Servings: 2

Ingredients:

2 cups cauliflower rice

1 cup cooked chicken breast, shredded

1/2 cup peas

2 tbsp olive oil

1 tsp garlic powder

Salt and pepper to taste

Preparation:

Get the olive oil heated in a skillet over medium heat. Add cauliflower rice and garlic powder, cooking for 3-4 minutes.

Stir in chicken and peas, cooking until heated through.

Season with salt and pepper before serving.

Nutritional Information (per serving):

Calories: 300 kcal

Protein: 30 g

Fat: 14 g

Carbohydrates: 14 g

Fibre: 5 g

Oxalates: 0 mg

Baked Salmon with Herbs

Servings: 2

Ingredients:

2 salmon fillets (6 oz each)

2 tbsp olive oil

1 tbsp lemon juice

1 tsp dill

Salt and pepper to taste

Preparation:

Preheat the oven to 375°F (190°C). Line a baking sheet with parchment paper.

Place salmon on the baking sheet and drizzle with olive oil and lemon juice.

Sprinkle dill, salt, and pepper on top.

Bake for about twenty minutes until cooked through and flaky.

Nutritional Information (per serving):

Calories: 350 kcal

Protein: 40 g

Fat: 20 g

Carbohydrates: 0 g

Fibre: 0 g

Oxalates: 0 mg

Chicken and Broccoli Casserole

Servings: 4

Ingredients:

2 cups cooked chicken, shredded

2 cups broccoli florets

1 cup cream of mushroom soup (low-sodium)

1 cup shredded mozzarella cheese

1/2 cup almond flour

Salt and pepper to taste

Preparation:

Preheat oven to 350°F (175°C).

In a large bowl, mix chicken, broccoli, soup, salt, and pepper.

Transfer to a baking dish and sprinkle mozzarella and almond flour on top.

Bake for 25-30 minutes until cheese is melted and bubbly.

Nutritional Information (per serving):

Calories: 400 kcal

Protein: 32 g

Fat: 24 g

Carbohydrates: 10 g

Fibre: 3 g

Oxalates: 0 mg

Stuffed Bell Peppers

Servings: 4

Ingredients:

4 bell peppers, halved and seeded

1 cup cooked quinoa

1 cup ground turkey, cooked

1 cup diced tomatoes

1 tsp Italian seasoning

1 cup mozzarella cheese, shredded

Preparation:

Preheat oven to 375°F (190°C). Get the pepper halves arranged in a baking dish.

In a bowl, mix quinoa, turkey, tomatoes, Italian seasoning, and half the cheese.

Fill pepper halves with the mixture and top with remaining cheese.

Cover with foil and bake for 30 minutes. Get the foil removed and bake for an additional 10 minutes until cheese is bubbly.

Nutritional Information (per serving):

Calories: 320 kcal

Protein: 25 g

Fat: 15 g

Carbohydrates: 24 g

Fibre: 6 g

Oxalates: 0 mg

Mediterranean Chickpea Salad

Servings: 2

Ingredients:

One can (15 oz) of rinsed and drained chickpeas

1/2 cucumber, diced

1/4 cup red onion, diced

1/4 cup parsley, chopped

2 tbsp olive oil

1 tbsp red wine vinegar

Salt and pepper to taste

Preparation:

In a large bowl, get the chickpeas, cucumber, onion, and parsley combined.

Drizzle with olive oil and vinegar, seasoning with salt and pepper.

Toss to combine and serve.

Nutritional Information (per serving):

Calories: 290 kcal

Protein: 12 g

Fat: 14 g

Carbohydrates: 36 g

Fibre: 10 g

Oxalates: 5 mg

Cabbage and Sausage Skillet

Servings: 4

Ingredients:

1 lb kielbasa sausage, sliced

4 cups green cabbage, chopped

1 onion, sliced

2 tbsp olive oil

Salt and pepper to taste

Preparation:

In a large skillet, get the olive oil heated over medium heat. Add sausage and cook until browned.

Add onion and cabbage, cooking until cabbage is tender.

Spice using salt and pepper before serving.

Nutritional Information (per serving):

Calories: 350 kcal

Protein: 20 g

Fat: 25 g

Carbohydrates: 12 g

Fibre: 4 g

Oxalates: 0 mg

Tuna Salad with Celery and Apples

Servings: 2

Ingredients:

1 can (5 oz) tuna, drained

1/4 cup celery, diced

1/4 cup apple, diced

2 tbsp mayonnaise

Salt and pepper to taste

Lettuce leaves for serving

Preparation:

In a bowl, mix tuna, celery, apple, mayonnaise, salt, and pepper.

Have it served on lettuce leaves or in a sandwich.

Nutritional Information (per serving):

Calories: 250 kcal

Protein: 22 g

Fat: 14 g

Carbohydrates: 10 g

Fibre: 2 g

Oxalates: 0 mg

Beef and Zucchini Stir-Fry

Servings: 2

Ingredients:

8 oz beef sirloin, sliced

1 cup zucchini, sliced

1/2 cup bell peppers, sliced

2 tbsp olive oil

2 tbsp soy sauce (gluten-free)

Salt and pepper to taste

Preparation:

Get olive oil heated in a skillet over medium heat. Add beef and cook until browned.

Get the zucchini and bell peppers added, cooking until tender.

Stir in soy sauce, and season with salt and pepper before serving.

Nutritional Information (per serving):

Calories: 350 kcal

Protein: 30 g

Fat: 22 g

Carbohydrates: 8 g

Fibre: 2 g

Oxalates: 0 mg

Chickpea and Spinach Curry

Servings: 2

Ingredients:

One can (15 oz) of rinsed and drained chickpeas

2 cups spinach, fresh

1 can (14 oz) coconut milk

2 tbsp curry powder

1 tbsp olive oil

Salt and pepper to taste

Preparation:

In a saucepan, have the olive oil heated over medium heat. Get the curry powder added and cook for 1 minute.

Stir in chickpeas and coconut milk, simmering for 10 minutes.

Add spinach and cook until wilted. Season with salt and pepper before serving.

Nutritional Information (per serving):

Calories: 300 kcal

Protein: 10 g

Fat: 20 g

Carbohydrates: 26 g

Fibre: 8 g

Oxalates: 0 mg

Chapter 5: Nourishing Dinners without Toxins

Herb-Roasted Chicken with Vegetables

Servings: 4

Ingredients:

4 chicken thighs (bone-in, skin-on)

2 cups carrots, chopped

2 cups zucchini, chopped

2 tbsp olive oil

1 tbsp rosemary, chopped

1 tbsp thyme, chopped

Salt and pepper to taste

Preparation:

Preheat oven to 400°F (200°C).

In a large bowl, toss chicken and vegetables with olive oil, rosemary, thyme, salt, and pepper.

Place on a baking sheet and roast for 35-40 minutes until chicken is cooked through.

Nutritional Information (per serving):

Calories: 380 kcal

Protein: 30 g

Fat: 24 g

Carbohydrates: 12 g

Fibre: 4 g

Quinoa Stuffed Bell Peppers

Servings: 4

Ingredients:

4 bell peppers, halved and seeded

1 cup quinoa, cooked

1 can (15 oz) black beans, drained and rinsed

1 cup corn (fresh or frozen)

1 tsp cumin

1 tsp paprika

Salt and pepper to taste

1 cup salsa

Preparation:

Preheat oven to 375°F (190°C).

In a bowl, combine cooked quinoa, black beans, corn, spices, and salsa.

Stuff each bell pepper half with the mixture and place in a baking dish.

Bake for about thirty minutes until peppers becomes tender.

Nutritional Information (per serving):

Calories: 280 kcal

Protein: 12 g

Fat: 4 g

Carbohydrates: 54 g

Fibre: 12 g

Salmon with Lemon-Dill Sauce

Servings: 4

Ingredients:

4 salmon fillets (6 oz each)

2 tbsp olive oil

2 tbsp fresh dill, chopped

1 lemon, zested and juiced

Salt and pepper to taste

Preparation:

Preheat oven to 375°F (190°C).

Place salmon on a baking sheet, drizzle with olive oil, lemon juice, salt, and pepper.

Bake for 15-20 minutes until cooked through.

Serve with lemon zest and dill on top.

Nutritional Information (per serving):

Calories: 360 kcal

Protein: 34 g

Fat: 22 g

Carbohydrates: 2 g

Fibre: 0 g

Zucchini Noodles with Pesto

Servings: 2

Ingredients:

2 medium zucchinis, spiralized

1/2 cup basil pesto (store-bought or homemade)

1 cup cherry tomatoes, halved

2 tbsp pine nuts, toasted

Salt and pepper to taste

Preparation:

In a skillet, lightly sauté zucchini noodles over medium heat for 2-3 minutes.

Add pesto and cherry tomatoes, stirring to combine, and heat for another minute.

Serve topped with pine nuts, salt, and pepper.

Nutritional Information (per serving):

Calories: 280 kcal

Protein: 6 g

Fat: 22 g

Carbohydrates: 18 g

Fibre: 4 g

Lentil Soup with Spinach

Servings: 4

Ingredients:

1 cup lentils, rinsed

4 cups vegetable broth

1 cup spinach, chopped

1 carrot, diced

1 onion, diced

2 garlic cloves, minced

1 tsp cumin

Salt and pepper to taste

Preparation:

In a large pot, sauté onion and garlic until soft.

Add carrots, lentils, broth, cumin, salt, and pepper.

Bring to a boil, then simmer for 30 minutes.

Stir in spinach and cook for an additional 5 minutes.

Nutritional Information (per serving):

Calories: 220 kcal

Protein: 14 g

Fat: 1 g

Carbohydrates: 38 g

Fibre: 12 g

Stuffed Eggplant with Quinoa and Feta

Servings: 4

Ingredients:

2 medium eggplants, halved and seeded

1 cup quinoa, cooked

1 cup cherry tomatoes, halved

1/2 cup feta cheese, crumbled

1 tbsp olive oil

Salt and pepper to taste

Preparation:

Preheat oven to 375°F (190°C).

Brush eggplant halves with olive oil, sprinkle with salt and pepper.

Roast in the oven for 20 minutes until soft.

In a bowl, combine quinoa, tomatoes, feta, and fill eggplant halves.

Bake for an additional 10 minutes.

Nutritional Information (per serving):

Calories: 300 kcal

Protein: 10 g

Fat: 14 g

Carbohydrates: 36 g

Fibre: 8 g

Beef Stir-Fry with Broccoli

Servings: 4

Ingredients:

1 lb beef sirloin, sliced thin

4 cups broccoli florets

2 tbsp soy sauce (gluten-free)

2 tbsp olive oil

2 garlic cloves, minced

1 tsp ginger, minced

Preparation:

Get the olive oil heated in a skillet over medium-high heat.

Add beef and cook until browned.

Add garlic, ginger, and broccoli, stir-frying until broccoli is tender.

Drizzle with soy sauce and serve.

Nutritional Information (per serving):

Calories: 350 kcal

Protein: 30 g

Fat: 20 g

Carbohydrates: 10 g

Fibre: 4 g

Baked Sweet Potatoes with Black Beans

Servings: 4

Ingredients:

4 medium sweet potatoes

1 can (15 oz) black beans, drained and rinsed

1 avocado, diced

1 tsp cumin

Salt and pepper to taste

Preparation:

Preheat oven to 400°F (200°C).

Bake sweet potatoes for 45-50 minutes until tender.

In a bowl, mix black beans, avocado, cumin, salt, and pepper.

Slice sweet potatoes open and fill with the black bean mixture.

Nutritional Information (per serving):

Calories: 400 kcal

Protein: 10 g

Fat: 7 g

Carbohydrates: 75 g

Fibre: 12 g

Mushroom Risotto

Servings: 4

Ingredients:

1 cup Arborio rice

4 cups vegetable broth

1 cup mushrooms, sliced

1/2 onion, diced

2 tbsp olive oil

1/4 cup parmesan cheese, grated

Salt and pepper to taste

Preparation:

Have the olive oil heated in a pot over medium heat.

Sauté onion and mushrooms until soft.

Add rice, stirring for 2-3 minutes.

Gradually add broth, one cup at a time, stirring until absorbed.

Stir in parmesan cheese, salt, and pepper before serving.

Nutritional Information (per serving):

Calories: 350 kcal

Protein: 10 g

Fat: 10 g

Carbohydrates: 60 g

Fibre: 3 g

Turkey Meatballs with Zucchini Noodles

Servings: 4

Ingredients:

1 lb ground turkey

1/2 cup breadcrumbs (gluten-free)

1 egg, beaten

1 tsp Italian seasoning

2 zucchinis, spiralized

2 cups marinara sauce

Preparation:

Preheat oven to 375°F (190°C).

In a bowl, mix turkey, breadcrumbs, egg, Italian seasoning, salt, and pepper.

Form into meatballs and place on a baking sheet.

Bake for 25 minutes until cooked through.

Serve over zucchini noodles with marinara sauce.

Nutritional Information (per serving):

Calories: 320 kcal

Protein: 25 g

Fat: 12 g

Carbohydrates: 24 g

Fibre: 4 g

Shrimp and Asparagus Stir-Fry

Servings: 2

Ingredients:

1 lb shrimp, peeled and deveined

2 cups asparagus, trimmed and cut into 2-inch pieces

2 tbsp olive oil

2 garlic cloves, minced

1 tbsp lemon juice

Salt and pepper to taste

Preparation:

Have the olive oil heated in a skillet over medium heat.

Add garlic and asparagus, stir-frying for 3 minutes.

Add shrimp and cook until pink and cooked through, about 5 minutes.

Drizzle with lemon juice before serving.

Nutritional Information (per serving):

Calories: 350 kcal

Protein: 30 g

Fat: 18 g

Carbohydrates: 10 g

Fibre: 4 g

Chickpea and Spinach Curry

Servings: 4

Ingredients:

One can (15 oz) of drained and rinsed chickpeas

2 cups spinach, chopped

1 can (14 oz) coconut milk

1 onion, diced

2 garlic cloves, minced

1 tbsp curry powder

Salt and pepper to taste

Preparation:

In a pot, sauté onion and garlic until they are soft.

Add curry powder, stirring for 1 minute.

Stir the chickpeas, coconut milk, salt, and pepper in.

Simmer for about fifteen minutes, then have the spinach added and cook until wilted.

Nutritional Information (per serving):

Calories: 320 kcal

Protein: 12 g

Fat: 15 g

Carbohydrates: 38 g

Fibre: 10 g

Baked Cod with Lemon and Herbs

Servings: 4

Ingredients:

4 cod fillets (6 oz each)

2 tbsp olive oil

2 tbsp lemon juice

1 tbsp parsley, chopped

Salt and pepper to taste

Preparation:

Preheat oven to 400°F (200°C).

Place cod on a baking sheet, drizzle with olive oil, lemon juice, salt, and pepper.

Bake for about fifteen minutes until fish can be easily flaked with a fork.

Garnish with parsley before serving.

Nutritional Information (per serving):

Calories: 280 kcal

Protein: 30 g

Fat: 14 g

Carbohydrates: 0 g

Fibre: 0 g

Vegetable Stir-Fry with Tofu

Servings: 4

Ingredients:

1 block (14 oz) firm tofu, cubed

4 cups mixed vegetables (bell peppers, broccoli, carrots)

2 tbsp soy sauce (gluten-free)

2 tbsp olive oil

2 garlic cloves, minced

Preparation:

Have the olive oil heated in a large skillet over medium heat.

Add tofu and cook until golden brown, about 5-7 minutes.

Add vegetables and garlic, stir-frying until tender.

Drizzle with soy sauce before serving.

Nutritional Information (per serving):

Calories: 280 kcal

Protein: 16 g

Fat: 16 g

Carbohydrates: 24 g

Fibre: 6 g

Cauliflower Fried Rice

Servings: 4

Ingredients:

1 head cauliflower, grated into rice-sized pieces

2 eggs, beaten

A cup of fresh or frozen peas and carrots

2 green onions, chopped

2 tbsp soy sauce (gluten-free)

2 tbsp olive oil

Preparation:

Have the olive oil heated in a skillet over medium heat.

Add cauliflower and cook for 5 minutes until tender.

Push cauliflower to one side, pour in beaten eggs, and scramble.

Mix in peas, carrots, green onions, and soy sauce. Cook for an additional 3 minutes.

Nutritional Information (per serving):

Calories: 220 kcal

Protein: 10 g

Fat: 10 g

Carbohydrates: 24 g

Fibre: 5 g

Chapter 7: Low-Oxalate Juices and Smoothies

Creamy Avocado Spinach Smoothie

Servings: 1

Ingredients:

1/2 ripe avocado

1 cup spinach leaves

1 cup unsweetened almond milk

1 banana

1 tbsp honey (optional)

Preparation:

In a blender, combine avocado, spinach, almond milk, banana, and honey.

Blend until smooth and creamy.

Pour into a glass and serve immediately.

Nutritional Information (per serving):

Calories: 280 kcal

Protein: 4 g

Fat: 14 g

Carbohydrates: 36 g

Fibre: 8 g

Refreshing Cucumber Melon Juice

Servings: 2

Ingredients:

1 medium cucumber, peeled and chopped

2 cups cantaloupe, cubed

1 tbsp lime juice

Mint leaves for garnish (optional)

Preparation:

In a blender, combine cucumber, cantaloupe, and lime juice.

Blend until smooth.

Strain through a fine-mesh sieve if desired.

Serve chilled, garnished with mint leaves.

Nutritional Information (per serving):

Calories: 80 kcal

Protein: 1 g

Fat: 0 g

Carbohydrates: 21 g

Fibre: 2 g

Pineapple Coconut Smoothie

Servings: 1

Ingredients:

1 cup fresh pineapple chunks

1/2 cup coconut milk (unsweetened)

1/2 cup ice

1/2 banana

Preparation:

In a blender, combine pineapple, coconut milk, ice, and banana.

Blend until smooth and creamy.

Pour into a glass and serve immediately.

Nutritional Information (per serving):

Calories: 220 kcal

Protein: 2 g

Fat: 8 g

Carbohydrates: 36 g

Fibre: 3 g

Sweet Carrot Ginger Juice

Servings: 2

Ingredients:

4 medium carrots, peeled and chopped

1-inch piece of fresh ginger, peeled

1 apple, cored and chopped

1 cup water

Preparation:

In a blender, combine carrots, ginger, apple, and water.

Blend until smooth.

Strain through a fine-mesh sieve if desired.

Serve chilled.

Nutritional Information (per serving):

Calories: 90 kcal

Protein: 1 g

Fat: 0 g

Carbohydrates: 22 g

Fibre: 3 g

Tropical Green Smoothie

Servings: 1

Ingredients:

1/2 cup frozen mango chunks

1/2 cup spinach leaves

1 cup coconut water

1 tbsp chia seeds

Preparation:

In a blender, combine mango, spinach, coconut water, and chia seeds.

Blend until smooth.

Pour into a glass and enjoy.

Nutritional Information (per serving):

Calories: 150 kcal

Protein: 3 g

Fat: 3 g

Carbohydrates: 30 g

Fibre: 5 g

Strawberry Banana Smoothie

Servings: 1

Ingredients:

1 cup fresh strawberries, hulled

1 banana

1 cup unsweetened almond milk

1 tbsp honey (optional)

Preparation:

In a blender, combine strawberries, banana, almond milk, and honey.

Blend until smooth and creamy.

Serve immediately.

Nutritional Information (per serving):

Calories: 180 kcal

Protein: 4 g

Fat: 3 g

Carbohydrates: 37 g

Fibre: 4 g

Zucchini Pineapple Juice

Servings: 2

Ingredients:

1 medium zucchini, chopped

1 cup pineapple chunks

1 cup water

1 tbsp lime juice

Preparation:

In a blender, combine zucchini, pineapple, water, and lime juice.

Blend until smooth.

Strain through a fine-mesh sieve if desired.

Serve chilled.

Nutritional Information (per serving):

Calories: 70 kcal

Protein: 1 g

Fat: 0 g

Carbohydrates: 18 g

Fibre: 2 g

Berry Almond Smoothie

Servings: 1

Ingredients:

1/2 cup mixed berries (blueberries, raspberries)

1/2 cup unsweetened almond milk

1/4 cup almond yoghourt

1 tbsp almond butter

Preparation:

In a blender, combine mixed berries, almond milk, almond yoghourt, and almond butter.

Blend until smooth.

Pour into a glass and serve immediately.

Nutritional Information (per serving):

Calories: 220 kcal

Protein: 6 g

Fat: 10 g

Carbohydrates: 30 g

Fibre: 5 g

Citrus Green Juice

Servings: 2

Ingredients:

2 cups kale leaves, stems removed

1 grapefruit, peeled and segmented

1 orange, peeled and segmented

1 cup water

Preparation:

In a blender, combine kale, grapefruit, orange, and water.

Blend until smooth.

Strain through a fine-mesh sieve if desired.

Serve chilled.

Nutritional Information (per serving):

Calories: 70 kcal

Protein: 2 g

Fat: 0 g

Carbohydrates: 17 g

Fibre: 3 g

Beet and Apple Smoothie

Servings: 1

Ingredients:

1/2 cup cooked beet, chopped

1 apple, cored and chopped

1/2 cup unsweetened almond milk

1 tbsp lemon juice

Preparation:

In a blender, combine beet, apple, almond milk, and lemon juice.

Blend until smooth.

Pour into a glass and enjoy.

Nutritional Information (per serving):

Calories: 130 kcal

Protein: 2 g

Fat: 3 g

Carbohydrates: 28 g

Fibre: 5 g

Kiwi Banana Smoothie

Servings: 1

Ingredients:

1 ripe kiwi, peeled and chopped

1 banana

1 cup coconut water

1 tbsp flaxseeds

Preparation:

In a blender, combine kiwi, banana, coconut water, and flaxseeds.

Blend until smooth.

Serve immediately.

Nutritional Information (per serving):

Calories: 180 kcal

Protein: 3 g

Fat: 2 g

Carbohydrates: 38 g

Fibre: 6 g

Minty Lime Cucumber Juice

Servings: 2

Ingredients:

1 large cucumber, peeled and chopped

1/4 cup fresh mint leaves

2 limes, juiced

1 cup water

Preparation:

In a blender, combine cucumber, mint, lime juice, and water.

Blend until smooth.

Strain through a fine-mesh sieve if desired.

Serve chilled.

Nutritional Information (per serving):

Calories: 30 kcal

Protein: 1 g

Fat: 0 g

Carbohydrates: 7 g

Fibre: 1 g

Mango Banana Smoothie

Servings: 1

Ingredients:

1 cup frozen mango chunks

1 banana

1 cup unsweetened almond milk

1/2 tbsp honey (optional)

Preparation:

In a blender, combine mango, banana, almond milk, and honey.

Blend until smooth.

Pour into a glass and serve immediately.

Nutritional Information (per serving):

Calories: 200 kcal

Protein: 3 g

Fat: 3 g

Carbohydrates: 46 g

Fibre: 4 g

Papaya Coconut Smoothie

Servings: 1

Ingredients:

1/2 cup papaya, cubed

1/2 cup coconut milk

1/2 banana

1 tbsp lime juice

Preparation:

In a blender, combine papaya, coconut milk, banana, and lime juice.

Blend until smooth.

Serve chilled.

Nutritional Information (per serving):

Calories: 210 kcal

Protein: 3 g

Fat: 7 g

Carbohydrates: 37 g

Fibre: 5 g

Almond Berry Juice

Servings: 1

Ingredients:

1/2 cup mixed berries (strawberries, blueberries)

1 cup unsweetened almond milk

1 tbsp almond butter

1/2 banana

Preparation:

In a blender, combine mixed berries, almond milk, almond butter, and banana.

Blend until smooth.

Pour into a glass and serve immediately.

Nutritional Information (per serving):

Calories: 220 kcal

Protein: 6 g

Fat: 10 g

Carbohydrates: 30 g

Fibre: 5 g

Chapter 8 – Bonus: 30-Day Low Oxalate Meal Plan

Day 1 to 7

Day 1

Breakfast: Savory Quinoa Porridge with Spinach and Eggs

Lunch: Grilled Chicken Salad with Cucumber and Feta

Dinner: Lemon Herb Grilled Salmon with Roasted Cauliflower

Snack: Coconut Yogurt with Fresh Berries

Juice/Smoothie: Tropical Green Smoothie

Day 2

Breakfast: Chia Seed Pudding with Coconut Milk

Lunch: Turkey Lettuce Wraps with Avocado

Dinner: Garlic Butter Shrimp with Zucchini Noodles

Snack: Apple Slices with Sunflower Seed Butter

Juice/Smoothie: Papaya Coconut Smoothie

Day 3

Breakfast: Scrambled Eggs with Bell Peppers and Onion

Lunch: Quinoa Salad with Grilled Veggies

Dinner: Baked Chicken Thighs with Brussels Sprouts

Snack: Homemade Trail Mix (pumpkin seeds, sunflower seeds)

Juice/Smoothie: Spinach and Cucumber Juice

Day 4

Breakfast: Smoothie Bowl with Coconut Flakes and Chia Seeds

Lunch: Beef Stir-Fry with Bell Peppers

Dinner: Stuffed Peppers with Ground Turkey and Rice

Snack: Celery Sticks with Hummus

Juice/Smoothie: Watermelon Mint Juice

Day 5

Breakfast: Egg Muffins with Spinach and Cheese

Lunch: Zucchini Noodles with Pesto Chicken

Dinner: Grilled Pork Chops with Asparagus

Snack: Carrot Sticks with Guacamole

Juice/Smoothie: Green Apple and Celery Juice

Day 6

Breakfast: Greek Yoghourt with Honey and Almonds

Lunch: Chicken Caesar Salad (no croutons)

Dinner: Roasted Duck Breast with Steamed Broccoli

Snack: Sliced Pear with Cheddar Cheese

Juice/Smoothie: Blueberry Almond Smoothie

Day 7

Breakfast: Cottage Cheese with Sliced Peaches

Lunch: Shrimp Salad with Avocado Dressing

Dinner: Baked Tilapia with Lemon and Herbs

Snack: Radish and Cucumber Slices

Juice/Smoothie: Orange Carrot Smoothie

Day 8 to 14

Day 8

Breakfast: Smoothie with Kale, Banana, and Almond Milk

Lunch: Grilled Vegetable and Chicken Wrap

Dinner: Beef and Broccoli Stir-Fry

Snack: Cherry Tomatoes with Feta

Juice/Smoothie: Strawberry Basil Smoothie

Day 9

Breakfast: Avocado Toast on Gluten-Free Bread

Lunch: Egg Salad Lettuce Wraps

Dinner: Lemon Garlic Chicken with Green Beans

Snack: Popcorn (air-popped, no butter)

Juice/Smoothie: Pineapple Spinach Smoothie

Day 10

Breakfast: Oatmeal with Almond Milk and Blueberries

Lunch: Chicken and Vegetable Soup

Dinner: Stuffed Acorn Squash with Quinoa

Snack: Almonds and Dried Cranberries

Juice/Smoothie: Cucumber Mint Smoothie

Day 11

Breakfast: Smoothie with Coconut Milk and Berries

Lunch: Zucchini and Tomato Salad

Dinner: Grilled Lamb Chops with Brussels Sprouts

Snack: Bell Pepper Strips with Hummus

Juice/Smoothie: Apple Ginger Juice

Day 12

Breakfast: Egg and Spinach Breakfast Wrap

Lunch: Grilled Salmon Salad with Avocado

Dinner: Chicken and Cauliflower Curry

Snack: Rice Cakes with Almond Butter

Juice/Smoothie: Berry Beet Smoothie

Day 13

Breakfast: Banana Chia Seed Pudding

Lunch: Turkey and Avocado Salad

Dinner: Roasted Chicken with Sweet Potatoes

Snack: Cucumber Slices with Cream Cheese

Juice/Smoothie: Watermelon Lime Juice

Day 14

Breakfast: Quinoa Breakfast Bowl with Nuts and Berries

Lunch: Beef and Vegetable Skewers

Dinner: Grilled Mahi Mahi with Asparagus

Snack: Trail Mix (nuts and seeds)

Juice/Smoothie: Spinach Mango Smoothie

Day 15 to 21

Day 15

Breakfast: Omelet with Mushrooms and Feta

Lunch: Chicken Salad with Grapes and Walnuts

Dinner: Pork Tenderloin with Green Beans

Snack: Hard-Boiled Eggs

Juice/Smoothie: Orange Mango Smoothie

Day 16

Breakfast: Smoothie Bowl with Coconut and Kiwi

Lunch: Lentil Salad with Roasted Vegetables

Dinner: Grilled Shrimp with Zucchini Noodles

Snack: Radishes with Hummus

Juice/Smoothie: Cucumber Lemonade

Day 17

Breakfast: Overnight Oats with Chia Seeds and Almonds

Lunch: Caesar Salad with Grilled Chicken

Dinner: Stuffed Bell Peppers with Turkey

Snack: Celery with Peanut Butter

Juice/Smoothie: Berry Citrus Smoothie

Day 18

Breakfast: Coconut Yogurt with Granola

Lunch: Quinoa Salad with Grilled Chicken

Dinner: Baked Cod with Mixed Vegetables

Snack: Mixed Nuts

Juice/Smoothie: Green Detox Smoothie

Day 19

Breakfast: Scrambled Eggs with Tomatoes and Spinach

Lunch: Tuna Salad with Avocado

Dinner: Roast Beef with Cauliflower Mash

Snack: Apple Slices with Cheese

Juice/Smoothie: Lemon Ginger Zinger

Day 20

Breakfast: Smoothie with Spinach, Mango, and Almond Milk

Lunch: Chickpea Salad with Cucumbers

Dinner: Grilled Chicken with Roasted Carrots

Snack: Popcorn with Nutritional Yeast

Juice/Smoothie: Blueberry Banana Smoothie

Day 21

Breakfast: Quinoa and Berry Bowl

Lunch: Grilled Chicken Wrap with Vegetables

Dinner: Pork Chops with Apples and Brussels Sprouts

Snack: Cucumber and Cream Cheese Bites

Juice/Smoothie: Strawberry Kiwi Smoothie

Day 22 to 30

Day 22

Breakfast: Oatmeal with Berries and Nuts

Lunch: Spinach Salad with Feta and Strawberries

Dinner: Baked Chicken Thighs with Cauliflower

Snack: Sliced Bell Peppers

Juice/Smoothie: Mango Coconut Smoothie

Day 23

Breakfast: Smoothie with Banana and Spinach

Lunch: Greek Salad with Grilled Chicken

Dinner: Lemon Garlic Shrimp with Broccoli

Snack: Mixed Nuts

Juice/Smoothie: Pineapple Kale Smoothie

Day 24

Breakfast: Cottage Cheese with Berries

Lunch: Chicken Lettuce Wraps with Avocado

Dinner: Baked Salmon with Green Beans

Snack: Carrot Sticks with Hummus

Juice/Smoothie: Green Apple Smoothie

Day 25

Breakfast: Quinoa Breakfast Bowl with Almond Milk

Lunch: Vegetable Stir-Fry with Tofu

Dinner: Grilled Steak with Cauliflower Rice

Snack: Cherry Tomatoes with Mozzarella

Juice/Smoothie: Watermelon Strawberry Juice

Day 26

Breakfast: Smoothie with Avocado and Banana

Lunch: Shrimp Salad with Avocado Dressing

Dinner: Stuffed Zucchini Boats

Snack: Rice Cakes with Nut Butter

Juice/Smoothie: Lemon Basil Smoothie

Day 27

Breakfast: Chia Seed Pudding with Coconut Milk

Lunch: Quinoa and Black Bean Salad

Dinner: Grilled Chicken with Spinach

Snack: Celery Sticks with Cream Cheese

Juice/Smoothie: Strawberry Mango Juice

Day 28

Breakfast: Scrambled Eggs with Zucchini

Lunch: Chicken Salad with Grapes and Walnuts

Dinner: Roasted Pork Loin with Vegetables

Snack: Hard-Boiled Eggs

Juice/Smoothie: Orange and Carrot Juice

Day 29

Breakfast: Smoothie Bowl with Banana and Spinach

Lunch: Lentil Soup with Vegetables

Dinner: Grilled Mahi Mahi with Asparagus

Snack: Sliced Cucumbers with Hummus

Juice/Smoothie: Berry Spinach Smoothie

Day 30

Breakfast: Quinoa Breakfast Bowl with Nuts and Berries

Lunch: Turkey Wrap with Lettuce and Avocado

Dinner: Baked Chicken with Brussels Sprouts

Snack: Mixed Nuts

Juice/Smoothie: Kiwi Pineapple Smoothie

Conclusion: A New Path to Wellness

As we conclude this journey through the world of low-oxalate living, it is vital to recognize the transformative potential of embracing a lifestyle that prioritises health and well-being. The insights and strategies shared in this book are designed not just as a dietary shift, but as a holistic approach to achieving optimal wellness. By understanding the impact of oxalates on our bodies and making conscious choices about what we consume, we can pave the way toward a life filled with abundant energy and reduced chronic pain.

Final Thoughts on Embracing a Low-Oxalate Lifestyle

Transitioning to a low-oxalate diet may initially seem daunting, but it is an empowering step toward reclaiming your health. Many individuals experience immediate benefits, including improved digestion, reduced inflammation, and increased energy levels. These changes often lead to a renewed sense of vitality and the ability to engage more fully in daily activities.

This journey is not just about eliminating high-oxalate foods but also about incorporating nourishing, low-oxalate alternatives that promote well-being. By embracing a variety of nutrient-dense foods, such as leafy greens, lean proteins, healthy fats, and vibrant fruits, you can create delicious and satisfying meals that support your body's needs. Over time, you may find yourself developing a deeper connection with the foods you consume and an appreciation for their role in your health journey.

Living with Abundant Energy and Without Chronic Pain

One of the most profound benefits of adopting a low-oxalate lifestyle is the potential to alleviate chronic pain and discomfort. Many people suffering from conditions such as kidney stones, fibromyalgia, and arthritis find that reducing oxalate intake leads to significant improvements in their symptoms. By prioritising low-oxalate foods, you can help minimise the risk of inflammation and promote overall body health.

Furthermore, a low-oxalate diet encourages a balanced intake of essential nutrients, which can improve energy levels and support mental clarity. With greater energy and reduced pain, individuals often experience a boost in motivation and enthusiasm for life, enabling them to pursue passions, hobbies, and relationships that may have previously felt out of reach.

Steps to Keep Your Health Thriving Long-Term

Sustaining a low-oxalate lifestyle requires commitment and mindfulness, but it is a journey that pays dividends in the form of long-term health. Here are several actionable steps to help ensure your continued wellness:

Educate Yourself: Continue to learn about oxalates and their effects on the body. Understanding the science behind your dietary choices can empower you to make informed decisions and explore new foods.

Plan Your Meals: Create a meal plan that incorporates a variety of low-oxalate foods. This not only helps to maintain dietary diversity but also reduces the temptation to revert to high-oxalate options.

Monitor Your Body's Response: Be mindful of how your body responds to various foods. Keeping a food diary can help you identify patterns and foods that may trigger discomfort, allowing you to adjust your diet accordingly.

Focus on Whole Foods: Focus on incorporating whole, minimally processed foods into your diet. These foods are often lower in oxalates and higher in essential nutrients, promoting overall health and well-being.

Seek Support: Surround yourself with a community of like-minded individuals who share your commitment to a low-oxalate lifestyle. Whether through online forums, social media groups, or local meet-ups, connecting with others can provide motivation and inspiration.

Consult Health Professionals: Consider working with a registered dietitian or healthcare provider who understands low-oxalate diets. They can offer personalised guidance and support as you navigate your dietary changes.

Practice Mindfulness: Incorporate mindfulness practices such as meditation or yoga to reduce stress, which can impact overall health. A calm mind fosters better food choices and promotes a healthier lifestyle.

Stay Hydrated: Adequate hydration is essential for flushing oxalates from the body and supporting kidney function. Aim for plenty of water throughout the day, particularly when consuming foods that may be higher in oxalates.

Experiment and Enjoy: Don't hesitate to try new recipes and foods. Embrace the culinary adventure of discovering delicious low-oxalate meals that excite your palate.

Listen to Your Body: Finally, be gentle with yourself. Everyone's journey is unique, and it's essential to listen to your body's cues as you adapt to a low-oxalate lifestyle.

By embracing these steps and committing to a low-oxalate lifestyle, you can create a new path to wellness that fosters abundant energy, reduced chronic pain, and a profound sense of well-being. The journey may have its challenges, but the rewards are immeasurable, offering you a vibrant, health-filled life.

4 BOOKS BONUS GIFTS

Please scan each QR code one by one, and you'll be directed to a website where you can claim your free books. Whenever you're prompted to enter a price, simply input "$0," as these books are completely free for you.

BONUS 2
50 JUICES

BONUS 3
50 SMOOTHIES

BONUS 4
50 SNACKS

BONUS 5
50 DESSERTS

Made in the USA
Columbia, SC
28 May 2025

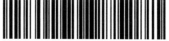

58615616R00059